Understanding
Yoga

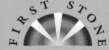

Contents

1 Introducing Yoga   4

The meaning of 'yoga'; Defining yoga; Science of yoga; Fundamental principles; Types of yoga (Hatha yoga; Iyengar yoga; Ashtanga vinyasa; Sivananda yoga; Tantra yoga; Karma yoga; Bhakti yoga; Jnana yoga; Raja yoga; Mantra yoga;); Dharma; Positive and negative.

2 A Brief History   12

Ancient history; Yoga today.

3 How It Works   16

Asanas; Skeletal structure; Circulatory system; Nervous system; Digestive system; Breath awareness; Breathing correctly; Abdominal breathing.

4 Who Can Benefit? 28

Back pain; Stress; Nervous conditions; Structural/
postural problems.

5 What To Expect From Yoga 32

Finding a practitioner; Preparing for classes; General
cautions; What to expect; Personal journey; Effort and
reward; Blocks to learning.

6 Practising Yoga 40

The eight limbs; Asana; Asana and the body-mind
connection; Practising asana; Principles of practice;
Breath and movement; Pranayama; Pranaya practice;
Chakras; Bandhas; Hasta mudras; Diet.

7 Relaxation 56

Stress; Physical relaxation; Mental relaxation; Spiritual
relaxation.

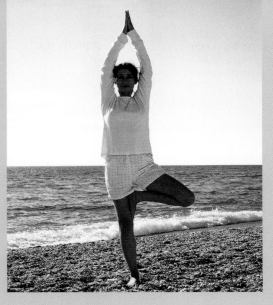

1

Introducing Yoga

Yoga is an Eastern practice that has long been popular in the Western world.

THE MEANING OF 'YOGA'

The Sanskrit term 'yoga' means 'to bind, attach and join; to yoke or unite body, mind and spirit; the disciplining of the intellect, mind, emotions and the will'.

A further meaning is 'to attain what was previously unattainable' or 'finding the means for bringing a desire into action'.

DEFINING YOGA

Yoga evolved in India long ago (see Chapter Two), but today its content is universal. Yoga is all about finding the means by which we can make the changes we desire in our lives.

Yoga is a system of education for mind, body and spirit. It is a holistic aid to the art of 'right' living. It deals with universal truths, and it is not linked to religion.

Yoga aims to provide a sense of unity with all in the world, using a system of techniques concerned with improving the

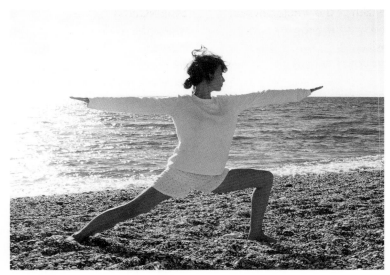

Yoga provides a sense of unity within ourselves and with the world around us.

health of the whole physical body, and all the systems within it. In turn, this acts as a means of improving mental and emotional states, taking control of the mind. In this way, it can be seen as an all-inclusive therapy, involving breath control, diet, relaxation, meditation, and physical exercises or movements (known as postures or asanas).

Used together, they form a powerful healing tool, helping to improve flexibility and to achieve a sense of calm and focus in the mind.

SCIENCE OF YOGA

The science of yoga begins with work on the physical body, which is, for most people, a good starting point.

When imbalance is felt at the physical level, the body's muscles, nerves and organs act in opposition to each other. Yoga aims to restore harmony and balance to bodily functions.

Another aspect of yoga is to do with focus. Yoga teaches us to act in such way that all our attention is directed towards the activity in which we are engaged, rather than thinking about something else. Yoga attempts to create a state in which we are always really present (focused to the present moment), in every action, in every moment. The advantage of this is that our performance is enhanced and we are conscious of our actions. Bringing together the mind, body and spirit towards self-realisation is the ultimate aim of yoga; to be united with the ultimate reality or final truth.

FUNDAMENTAL PRINCIPLES

Yoga ultimately seeks to liberate us from our basic perception of who we are, and our obsession of identifying ourselves with our possessions, body, mind, and relationships.

The teachings of yoga aim to help us understand that we are beyond this – from a yogic perspective we are super-conscious, unlimited and free.

TYPES OF YOGA

Each person has different strengths, weaknesses, emotional needs and mental capacities. Yoga has different approaches so that everyone can practise it. Most popular classes in the west include hatha yoga postures or asanas.

- **Hatha yoga:** The broad term for classical yoga postures (asanas), breathing and relaxation techniques. It is strengthening and toning for the body and aims at uniting body and mind.

- **Iyengar yoga:** This includes postures based on hatha yoga. It is a precise and physically demanding form of yoga, incorporating props and Iyengar teachings.

- **Ashtanga vinyasa:** This incorporates postures with ujai breathing in a flowing sequence. It aims to create

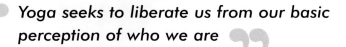

Yoga seeks to liberate us from our basic perception of who we are

heat in the body to release toxins and increase focus, strength and stamina.

- **Sivananda yoga:** With hatha-based postures, sivananda offers spiritual teaching, chanting, meditation, and breathing exercises.
- **Tantra yoga:** This aims to liberate through ritual visualisation, subtle energy work, and perception of identity of the ordinary and transcendental worlds.
- **Karma yoga:** Action through self-transcending service – work for others for no material gain.
- **Bhakti yoga:** Also known as devotional yoga, this teaches surrender in the face of the divine.
- **Jnana yoga:** This liberates through applying higher wisdom, discerning between the real and unreal.
- **Raja yoga:** Liberates through meditation and advanced concentration, involving the eight-fold path of Patanjali.
- **Mantra yoga:** As its name suggests, this liberates through 'yoga of potent sound' – recitation of mantra.

DHARMA

All forms of yoga provide guidance in leading a sound moral life – the 'dharma' (meaning morality, law and virtue) observes practising compassion (karuna), chastity (bramacharya), kindness (maitri), truthfulness (satya), non-theft (asteya), and non-harming (ahimsa).

POSITIVE AND NEGATIVE

A morally sound life helps us to stop creating negative effects, so that we can realise our true nature. The repeated practice of exercises or techniques of yoga produces a positive response, but the practice of letting go of old patterns of behaviour and attachments is just as important – it reveals the true mind.

Yoga aims to be a process of replacing our unconscious patterns of behaviour with new. In yoga, no effort is ever wasted. Any attempt at transforming ourselves makes a difference.

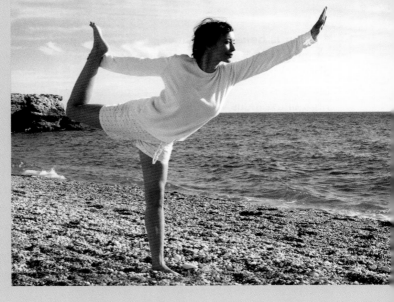

2

A Brief History

Yoga is believed to have originated in India about 5,000 years ago.

Engravings in stone depict yogis of the Indus Valley civilisation (2,500-1,800 BC), a pre-Vedic culture.

ANCIENT HISTORY

With the invasion by Indo-Aryan tribes from the north, hermit-like sages evolved, seeking life's truth from within. The first written accounts of their knowledge were written by the Vedas, which later came to constitute the *Upanishads*.

The Vedic scriptures offered a path of life. They were written by seers, who were regarded as accomplished mystics.

The *Upanishads* (600-400 BC) contain some of yoga's most important literary works, the *Bhagavad-Gita*, a treatise, looks at the central yogic precept of non-attachment to material things, with a section on yoga theory. Patanjali's yoga sutras enumerate the eight stages of yoga (the eight limbs), systemizing an approach to yoga. This was followed by *Hathayogapradipika,* which describes how to practise postures, cleansing and breathing techniques.

YOGA TODAY

Yoga is very much part of a spiritual heritage from the past being reclaimed today. Yogic practices give direct benefits to everyone – regardless of their spiritual aims.

Mental and physical therapy is one of yoga's important achievements, working on holistic principles of harmony and unification makes it powerful and effective.

Research shows Yoga has succeeded as an alternative form of therapy in helping people with asthma, blood pressure problems, diabetes, digestive disorders, arthritis and other chronic ailments. Most people, however, use yoga as a way of maintaining health and well-being in an increasingly stressful society.

Yoga gives people a means to find their own way of connecting with their true selves.

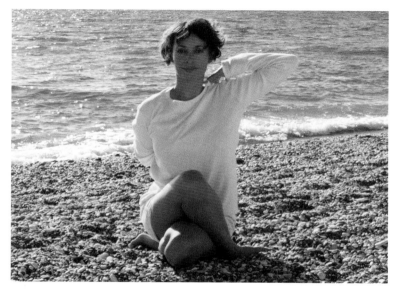

Yoga remains as relevant to health and well-being today as it did when it was first practised by the ancient Vedic seers.

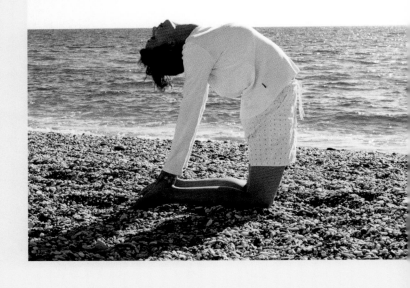

3

How It Works

Yoga postures are designed to cleanse, tone and purify the whole body, which, in turn, affects the mind, improving stamina, strength, and balance.

Yoga combines correct breathing (yogic breathing) with yoga asanas (postures) to affect all parts of the body, including the spine, glands and internal organs.

ASANAS
The asanas work on more than one physical aspect at a time, helping to improve everything from blood circulation and nerve function, to digestive and eliminative systems.

Each asana can have a massaging or squeezing effect on a gland or organ; at the same time, everything is linked via the spinal cord to the brain. Positive effects on the glands and nerves produce a positive, healthy, emotional state of being. When practising asanas, our metabolic rates slow down, as does our consumption of oxygen. In

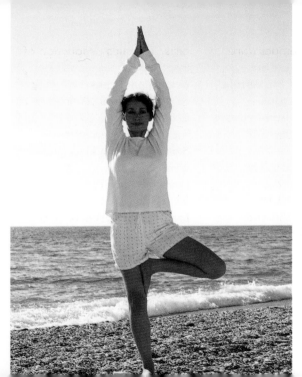

Practising various asanas, such as the tree pose (vrkasana), not only helps to improve body tone and posture, but it also has a positive effect on emotional well-being.

addition, body temperature drops (the opposite effect to what happens during 'normal' forms of exercise), altering electro-chemical activity in the nervous system.

SKELETAL STRUCTURE

Yoga postures help get rid of rigidity within the body. The postures stretch muscles deeply, and, as the muscles loosen and stretch, so do the ligaments that hold the bones in place. The stretching effect on the muscles and joints stimulate the skin and muscle cells. This aids production of lubrication fluid in the joints, helping the bones to realign.

CIRCULATORY SYSTEM

Blood circulation is improved through performing the asanas and breathing exercises.

Yoga teaches the individual to become more aware of breathing and use of the lungs. Breathing deeply and correctly allows oxygenated blood to be pumped more effectively to the organs, helping to carry away toxins.

NERVOUS SYSTEM

The nervous and endocrine (hormonal) systems are affected through the spinal nerve centre. Yoga helps to control and release nervous energy.

DIGESTIVE SYSTEM

The stretching and massaging action some poses perform on the internal organs, such as back and forward bends and twist postures (see pages 25-27), help the digestive system to function at peak efficiency.

BREATH AWARENESS

Breath awareness is an important part of yoga practice. Breathing can be used as a focus point, as well as helping to release and relax body and mind. This has a general positive effect on an individual's health, strengthening the lungs and the muscles used for breathing.

Oxygen is essential to life to create energy. Breathing supplies oxygen to all the cells of the body, removing carbon dioxide and toxins from the blood and improving

INVERTED POSTURES

Inverted postures reverse the action of gravity in the body and turn everything upside down mentally. They allow a rich supply of blood to the brain, nourishing neurones and cells, and positively influencing the pituitary gland.

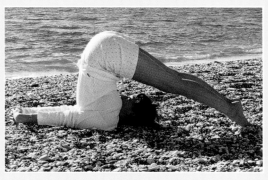

The plough (halasana) can help regulate the activity of the thyroid gland and stimulate the thymus gland, boosting the immune system.

The plough (halasana) helps increase flexibility in the cervical region of the spine, stretching and strengthening the muscles of the back, shoulders, abdomen and arms, while benefiting the circulatory system.

circulation. A loss of oxygen means a loss of mental balance, concentration and emotional control.

For most people, 'normal' breathing expels and replaces only about two-thirds of the air in the lungs. In our stressful society, many people breathe from the top part of their lungs only. This is shallow breathing, and it is a sign of stress and anxiety. Shallow breathing starves the body of essential oxygen and prevents complete elimination of noxious waste.

Yogic and pranayama breathing exercises help you to increase the depth and control of your breath. This has a direct effect on the mind, linking body, mind and breath, benefiting you as a whole.

CORRECT BREATHING AND ABDOMINAL BREATHING

Correct breathing demands a three-part movement.

Firstly, the diaphragm causes the abdomen to expand, filling the lower lungs.

Next, the intercostal muscles expand the ribcage and fill the middle lungs.

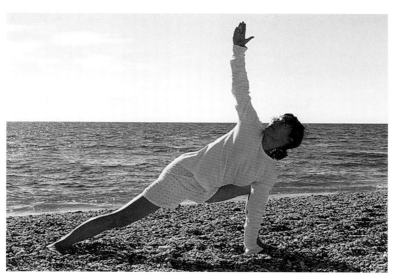

It is important to breathe correctly, and not to 'hold' the breath, when performing all yoga asanas.

Finally, the collarbone lifts slightly to bring air to the top of the lungs; focus on keeping the exhalation smooth and slow.

ABDOMINAL BREATHING

Abdominal breathing forms an important first step in yoga practice, making proper use of the diaphragmatic muscle at the base of the lungs.

Lying flat on your back in the savasana corpse pose, you can become far more aware of your breath. Learn how to breathe through your nose, using your diaphragm to draw air into the lowest and largest part of the lungs. Breathing correctly, the abdomen rises on inhalation and sinks on exhalation.

BACKBENDS

Backbend postures turn the body out to face the world. They invigorate and stimulate, expanding the chest and encouraging inhalation, and are associated with the attitude of embracing life. They counter gravity, so they require strength.

The bow posture helps to bring elasticity to the spine and tones the abdominal organs. It creates a feeling of openness, helping to improve posture and encourage suppleness. The bow pose can help improve hunching of the thoracic area of the spine and relieve some chest ailments.

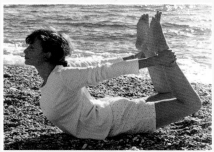

The bow pose (dhanurasana) helps to improve posture and suppleness.

FORWARD BENDS

Forward bending postures are passive movements in which gravity is used to stretch the muscles, strengthen the spine, release tension and pain, and encourage relaxation.

In a forward bend, the whole spinal column is toned, while the abdominal organs and heart are massaged. This posture can help the action of the kidneys and digestion and circulation, as well as toning the sexual organs.

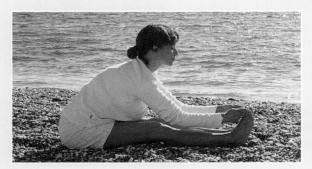

The forward bend (pashmottinasana) tones the spinal column.

SPINAL TWISTS

The twist series of postures help to make the spinal column more flexible. They also encourage the abdominal muscles to stretch and compress, massaging internal organs, such as the pancreas, kidneys, stomach and small intestines.

The spinal twist gives a lateral stretch to the back muscles and hips. This posture can increase synovial fluid to the joints, helping to tone the spinal nerves, muscles and the sympathetic nervous system.

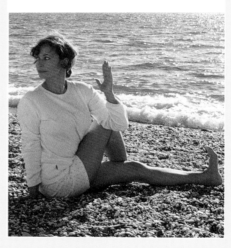

The sitting spinal twist (ardha matsyendrasana) encourages flexibility.

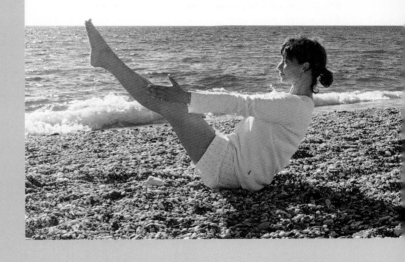

4

Who Can Benefit?

People of all ages and ability can benefit from yoga.

In order to maximise the benefits, it is important to find the right teacher, the correct type of yoga and the appropriate level (see pages 8-11).

In fact, people with specific needs – pregnant women, those with disabilities, ME and MS sufferers – can often find specialist teachers and classes. People with ailments of all kinds will find that yoga helps them.

BACK PAIN

Yoga can help those suffering back, shoulder and neck problems.

Where back pain is due to stress or minor injury, yoga can help to release back-muscle spasm through relaxation and awareness.

STRESS

Yoga can give relief from pain and stress-related problems.

Physical and mental tension often aggravates many ailments. Stress affects our muscles, joints and ligaments, which leads to fatigue and body aches. Stress can also cause overstimulation of the mind, which can lead to insomnia and nervous disorders. In turn, this can negatively affect the immune system.

Yoga helps the individual to relax, release and so gain control of dealing with stress.

The yoga pupil will learn how to release stress in a positive manner, which is invaluable for preventing illness.

NERVOUS CONDITIONS

Yoga helps those suffering from conditions that are related to imbalance in the nervous system. This includes headaches and migraine, asthma, tension, depression and anxiety.

STRUCTURAL/POSTURAL PROBLEMS

People with postural problems, stiff hips, collapsed chests and curvature of the spine, will all benefit from yoga.

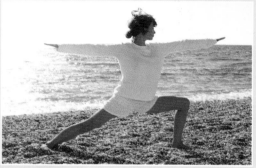

STANDING POSTURES

Standing postures have a stretching, strengthening effect throughout the body. They are very useful for people who sit down a lot and suffer from stiffness or pain in the back. They also help increase oxygenation and lung capacity.

Standing postures, such as the warrior pose (virabhadrasana), work to strengthen and tone the legs, relieve cramp in the calf and thigh muscles, and help to tone the arms, back, chest and abdominal organs.

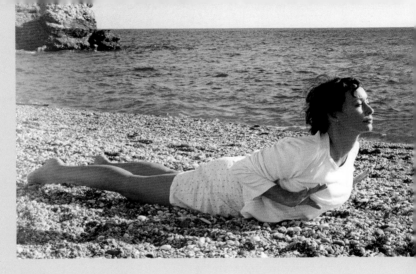

5 What To Expect
From Yoga

For those new to yoga, there are a whole host of questions that may need answering, usually about finding a practitioner, what to expect from classes, and how long it will take before the benefits can be felt.

FINDING A PRACTITIONER
Look for a well-qualified yoga tutor (see page 61) who is well aware of the guidelines about teaching yoga safely, such as using aids like blocks and belts if necessary.

Always let your tutor know about any medical conditions or injuries you have, so they can give you the best advice and provide you with alternative work or modifications if necessary.

Yoga is perfectly safe when practised correctly and mindfully under the supervision of a qualified teacher.

PREPARING FOR CLASSES
Always wear comfortable, non-restrictive clothing for yoga sessions.

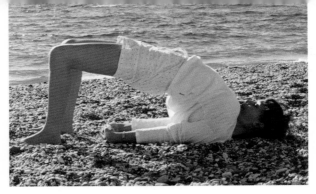

The bridge pose (setu bandhasana) is generally strengthening, toning the thighs, arms, achilles tendon and spinal region.

For the various exercises, you should always use a non-slip mat and practise in your bare feet. Some yoga classes will provide mats, but if in doubt, ask your tutor before your first class.

Always practise yoga on an empty stomach – about two to three hours after food, and about one hour after a drink.

GENERAL CAUTIONS

Consult your doctor or a yoga specialist if you are uncertain about a technique or your initial level of health and fitness. You should always see your doctor before beginning yoga if any of the following apply to you:

- Any health problem
- Any kind of surgery
- Any kind of injury
- Pregnancy.

WHAT TO EXPECT

Yoga is a non-competitive activity. Often, there will be a mixture of abilities in a class, working at different levels towards the same goal. An experienced tutor will balance classes so that everyone is able to gain some reward.

You may be surprised at how gentle yoga seems at first, but do not let this fool you. Although yoga exercises muscles in a different way to more traditional forms of exercise, it will still help you to develop a strong, flexible, svelte physique. It can also be practised as a complement to weight training, other sports or aerobic work.

Few sports demand that you lie down and relax, but be prepared for this in yoga classes. You will learn about breath awareness, and breathing techniques and exercises (pranayama).

PERSONAL JOURNEY

People new to yoga often ask, "How long will it take before I see results?"

It is best to see yoga as a journey. It is important to realise that each individual has a different level of ability and different needs. For each person, there will be a unique timescale of development, dependent on many aspects, including initial level of fitness, flexibility, structure, co-ordination, and ability to relax and breathe. People with injuries and medical conditions may take longer to adapt.

Most people feel some benefit even from their first yoga class. Following this, you may notice a series of changes at different times. For example, you may feel more relaxed, energised and toned initially, but, after a while, you may realise you are more aware of correct posture and so you may start adjusting your standing or sitting position automatically.

I have found that most newcomers to yoga generally experience a better and deeper sleep, feeling more refreshed and focused during the day.

Most people that practise yoga regularly find that it provides a means for them to release and control stress. Others feel benefits from improved posture, body and breath awareness and increased ability to relax.

EFFORT AND REWARD

The results you reap from yoga are down to you. The progress you make is directly related to what you want to put in. For example, you could decide to practise yoga once or twice a day, or once a week.

You may decide to look deeper into the philosophy behind yoga and gain extra knowledge from books, courses or yogis. The choice of how far you go, and how you use yoga in your life, is up to you.

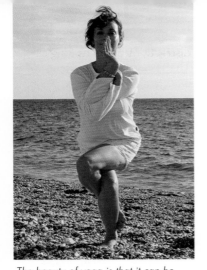

The beauty of yoga is that it can be adapted to fit in with almost any lifestyle and level of ability. However, it is worth remembering that you get out what you put in.

BLOCKS TO LEARNING

As recognised in the *Bhagavad-Gita* "the self can be the self's worst enemy".

Patanjali, the sage who wrote *Patanjali's Yoga Sutras* (one of the first known written scripts systemising yoga as one of the steps to enlightenment), states that there are nine hindrances that may arise in the discipline of practicing yoga. He lists these as:

• Sickness
• Apathy

- Doubt
- Heedlessness
- Sloth
- Dissipation
- False vision
- Non-attainment of the stages of yoga
- Instability.

These are mainly self-inflicted limitations. It also mentions in the *Yoga-Bhashya* literature that distractions occur as long as one of the five types of mental fluctuations are present – when the mind either perceives, misperceives, imagines, remembers, or is asleep.

When the mind can be controlled, the hindrances can be removed. Yoga seeks to take control of the mind by developing focus and 'one-pointedness' of the mind.

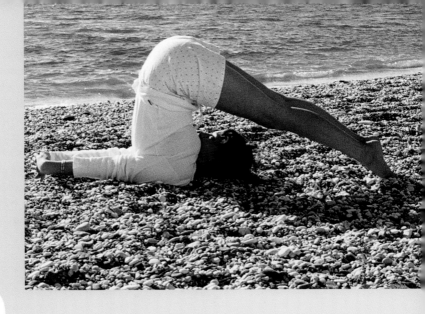

6 Practising Yoga

We have discovered that yoga is a personal journey. It can be broken down into different stages.

THE EIGHT LIMBS

The eight limbs or stages of yoga are based on Patanjali's yoga sutras. These describe the steps along the path to self-realisation, and all stages should be observed and practised to help bring together mind, body and spirit.

The eight stages are:

❶ **Yama (abstention):** Yoga students should practise non-violence, truthfulness, non-stealing, non-possessiveness, and control of sexual energy.

❷ **Niyama (observances):** This refers to austerity, purity, contentment, study, and the surrender of ego.

❸ **Asana (steady poses):** See page 42.

❹ **Pranayama (rhythmic control of the breath):** Yoga students will need to practise breathing exercises.

❺ **Pratyahara (sense control):** Referred to as

41

'the limb of steadiness', this stage brings the mind back to the rhythm of breath, calming and controlling the mind and developing focus.

❻ Dharana (concentration): Yoga students will learn how to control and apply their concentration.

❼ Dhyana (meditation): In Dhyana, it is said that 'yoga leads to meditation, helping us to create inner peace'.

❽ Samadi (super-consciousness): This refers to the culmination of the stages of yoga, where the student achieves a superconscious state.

ASANA

Asana is spoken of as the first part of Hatha yoga (see page 9).

Asana practice involves body postures, or exercises. They should be practised properly, with alertness, without tension, and in a relaxed state, using the breath to help relax and focus the individual.

When performing the asanas the body resembles the forms of many different creatures and legendary heroes. The names of the asanas are significant and illustrate the principle of evolution.

Some asanas are named after vegetation, such as 'the tree' (see page 45) and 'lotus'. Others are named after insects, including 'the locust' and 'the scorpion'. Some asanas take their names from aquatic and amphibious creatures, such as 'the fish' and 'the crocodile', as well as reptiles ('the cobra'), birds ('the peacock' and 'the swan'),

Having done asana, one attains steadiness of body and mind, freedom from disease, and lightness of limbs.
Hatha Yoga Pradipika

and mammals ('the dog', 'the cat' and 'the camel').

ASANA AND THE BODY-MIND CONNECTION

Patanjali described yoga as the "science of the mind". Our state of mind is all-important, ultimately affecting everything that we do.

The body and mind are not separate, but connected. The gross form is the body, the subtle form is the mind. Asana integrates and harmonises the two.

The body and mind can create mental and physical tensions or knots. Every mental knot has a corresponding physical, muscular knot, and vice versa.

Asana practice can release these physical and mental tensions by dealing with them on a physical level, acting through the body to influence the mind and helping to release dormant energy.

To take control of the mind, the yoga student must control stress. In this way yoga can be a major key to finding happiness.

BALANCING POSTURES

Balancing postures help to improve co-ordination, inducing physical balance, which acts to still unconscious movement. The focus required to perform the balancing moves develops concentration on an emotional, mental and psychic level. This helps to balance the nervous system and remove stress and anxiety.

The tree pose (vrkasana) helps to develop concentration, improves physical balance and posture, while toning the leg muscles.

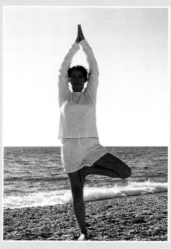

The tree pose (vrkasana) is a balancing posture that helps to improve co-ordination.

PRACTISING ASANA

As a relaxed body and mind function more efficiently, asana practice should start and finish with relaxation.

A balanced yoga asana class will include breath awareness and limbering, followed by moving the spine in all directions through use of appropriate postures and counterposes, starting with the easiest, working up to the more advanced, and back down to relaxation.

When you start practising yoga and go into a posture or movement that feels tense, it is hard to notice anything else but that tension. This may put you off practising yoga at first, but it is simply that you are trying to do something too advanced for your current level. You should start at the correct level of class for you, i.e. beginners. Accepting the level you are at is all-important to finding the qualities essential to practise asana. Recognise your own starting point, practise the breathing and postures progressively, and you will find more steadiness, comfort and overall alertness.

A good teacher will help you to practise the appropriate exercises for your level of ability and ensure that you practise the exercises in a balanced manner.

PRINCIPLES OF PRACTICE

In yoga, it is important to co-ordinate your movements with your breathing. You should breathe slowly and deeply, through your nose, going in to and coming out of each position slowly, staying relaxed.

As yoga is non-competitive, do not try to achieve what you cannot do – there is no gain with strain in yoga. The aim is to remain mentally relaxed while stretching and strengthening your physical body. The more relaxed you are, the easier it will be to perform asanas.

BREATH AND MOVEMENT

The quality of our breath is very important, as it expresses our inner feelings. The breath is the link between the inner and outer body, and it is only by bringing the breath and mind into unison that we realise the true quality of an asana. The first step of yoga practice is to allow every movement to be led by breath. The simple exercise of raising the arms as you inhale and lowering them as you exhale will help you to find the rhythm of combined breath and movement.

PRANAYAMA

'Prana' means 'life force' and 'yama' means 'control'. 'Pranayama' is generally termed as 'breath control', incorporating various breathing exercises.

The purpose of pranayama is to understand and control breathing and the pranic process in the body, as the way we breathe affects our whole being. Pranayama aims to remove impurities from the body so that the mind can become clear and focused.

The process of breathing is also linked to the brain via the hypothalmus, affecting the central nervous system. When nerve impulses are rhythmic

SIDEWAYS STRETCHES

These postures help to stretch and tone the muscles of the arms and legs, strengthening the internal organs and improving your concentration and sense of balance.

The triangle pose affects the muscles at the sides of the trunk, the waist, and the backs of the legs. It also strengthens the pelvic area, improving the strength and flexibility of the hip joint, while toning the reproductive organs.

This pose also stimulates the nervous system and helps to improve digestion. It activates intestinal peristalsis, which helps to alleviate constipation.

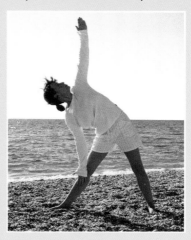

and steady, so are the brain waves. Erratic breathing creates disturbed responses.

PRANAYAMA PRACTICE
In pranayama practices there are four aspects of breathing:
- Inhalation
- Exhalation
- Internal breath retention
- External breath retention.

Perhaps the most important part of pranayama is breath retention (khumbhaka), but in order to practise this successfully, there must be a gradual development of control over respiration.

Initially, emphasis is given to inhalation and exhalation, to strengthen the lungs and balance the nervous and pranic systems. This prepares the body for the practice of retention. It is important to learn pranayama under the guidance of an experienced teacher.

CHAKRAS
On a physical level, chakras are associated with the main nerve plexus and endocrine

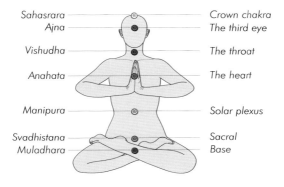

THE CHAKRAS

Sahasrara	Crown chakra
Ajna	The third eye
Vishudha	The throat
Anahata	The heart
Manipura	Solar plexus
Svadhistana	Sacral
Muladhara	Base

Chakras are part of the Indian yogic philosophy and are used to concentrate the mind during yoga practice.

(hormone-regulating) glands in the body. Chakras are part of the Indian yogic philosophy. There are believed to be seven chakras or 'wheels of energy' (see page 51). Each has a corresponding colour, a sound perception, and a biological function. Chakras may be used as focus points on which to direct the mind to improve a particular yoga practice.

BANDHAS

The Sanskrit term 'bandha' means 'to lock' or 'to hold' or 'tighten'. This precisely describes the physical action involved with bandhas in yoga practice. The aim is to lock vital energy, through yogic breathing, into particular areas of the body. It is used at a higher yogic level to awaken psychic faculties.

On a physical level, bandha works to support the body in the practice of yoga exercises. Bandha helps to strengthen the associated muscles and also tones the visceral organs, muscles, nerves and glands.

There are three types of bandha:

- **Moola bandha:** The technique where some of the muscles of the pelvic floor are contracted and held.
- **Uddiyana bandha:** This concerns contraction of the abdominal muscles, both inward and upward.
- **Jalandhara bandha:** This is known as the throat lock where the head is bent forward so the chin presses the neck.

Bandhas are practised combined with asana exercises.

HASTA MUDRAS

Hasta mudras are the hand gestures used in yoga practice. They help to strengthen, purify, calm and concentrate the student, enhancing energy flow. They can also be used in meditation and pranayama breathing practices.

DIET

Diet plays an important part in the yogic process. The yogic scriptures divide food into three types:

- **Sattvic (pure):** Sattvic foods increase strength, purity, health and joy, bringing purity and calmness to the mind. They are seen as soothing and nourishing to the body, helping to improve mental clarity. These foods include pure fruit juices, fresh and dried fruits, nuts and berries, legumes, raw or lightly cooked vegetables, salads, seeds, wholegrains, fresh herbs and dairy products. A sattvic diet supplies maximum energy, increasing vitality and strength.

- **Rajasic (stimulating):** Rajasic foods tend to be bitter, sour, salty, pungent or hot. A yogic diet avoids rajasic or overstimulating foods, such as onions, garlic, coffee, tea, ready-prepared convenience foods, refined sugar and soft drinks. These foods can cause a restless state of mind, leading to hyperactivity, and destroy the body-mind balance.

- **Tamasic (impure or rotten):** These foods are considered stale, tasteless, putrid, impure or rotten. Meat, fish, eggs, alcohol and drugs are all tamasic. Other tamasic foods include anything that has been burnt, fried, barbecued or reheated. Tamasic foods are avoided in the yogic diet because they produce feelings of heaviness and lethargy.

Yogis believe that a person's food preference reflects their level of mental purity. Over time, as the individual develops spiritually, their tastes will alter.

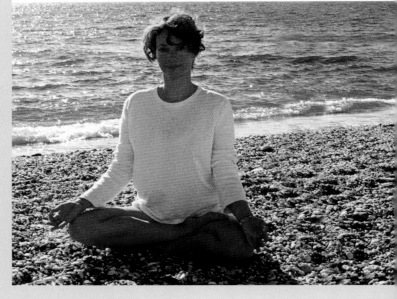

7

Relaxation

Being able to relax is important for everyone – in the course of their everyday life as well as for yoga practice.

Relaxation is a natural way of recharging body and mind. It is necessary for good health and for peace of mind.

STRESS

All action creates a type of stress. Some can be useful, helping us to perform to the best of our abilities, but undue tensions wear down our body and mind. Many aspects of modern life make it increasingly difficult to relax, and many people unknowingly waste large amounts of energy.

The physiology of action shows that stimulation is taken in through the senses. Then nerve impulses are sent via the nervous system to the mind. When analysing the stimuli, the mind decides what action is to be taken and then sends an impulse to the muscles. This involves extra supplies of energy, so that the action can be performed by muscle contraction. This process in itself means we are constantly using energy. A key to relaxation is to reduce the number of stimuli to which we are subjected.

PHYSICAL RELAXATION

Many people find that they have trained their muscles to be tense, keeping them in a state of readiness and wasting energy. Yoga asana techniques retrain the muscles to relax, and many people find that they have a deeper, more refreshing sleep.

MENTAL RELAXATION

Our minds are constantly bombarded with stimuli, overloading and exhausting it. Thinking, worrying and tension use up large amounts of energy, often more than required for physical work.

The mind needs to unwind and recoup its energies, and time needs to be set aside to do this or mental fatigue can set in, which affects the physical body. Yogic breathing exercises help to develop mental calmness, using the power of thought to achieve inner peace, with physical relaxation following mental relaxation.

SPIRITUAL RELAXATION
Tuning to a higher or divine source can bring complete mental and physical relaxation. This brings the realisation that all happiness comes from within.

Yoga provides techniques for this inner tuning, enabling us to break down the boundaries that separate us from others and our inner self.

It is often said that yoga leads to meditation, preparing the body to sit comfortably for long stretches of time. For most people, the mind jumps from thought to thought constantly, using large amounts of energy. Meditation helps to focus the mind. A feeling of oneness, absolute silence and peace can be experienced, giving a profound inner relaxation to the body and mind and deeply relieving stress.

For yoga relaxation and meditation exercises, see page 60.

RELAXATION & MEDITATION

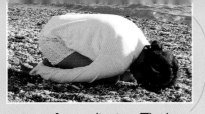

One of the main aims of practising yoga is to help increase your ability to relax through breathing and practising the postures. Relaxation techniques are also included in yoga classes, usually in the savasana corpse pose; when lying on your back you completely let go of tension through instruction or visualisation.

The well-known half or full lotus pose (ardha padmasana – see page 56) enables the body to be held steady for long periods, making it an ideal posture for meditation. The legs form a tripod for a firm base and an upright spine – allowing an enhanced flow of prana energy to the chakras. The posture has a relaxing, toning effect on the nervous system, stimulating the digestive process.

The child's pose (above) is a relaxation posture used for relaxing the whole psycho-physiological system between practising more demanding asanas.

Further Information

Yoga is taught all over the world, by private teachers working from home, as well as in clinics, educational institutions, health clubs and yoga centres.

You can find out about the main governing body of each country by investigating on the internet.

YOGA IN THE UK

The British Wheel of Yoga is the governing body of yoga in the UK, endorsed and supported by the Sports Council.

The British Wheel Of Yoga,
Central Office,
25 Jermyn Street,
Sleaford,
Lincolnshire,
NG34 7RU.
Tel: 01529 306851
Fax: 01529 303233
Email: information@bwy.org.uk
Website: www.bwy.org.uk

About the author

Belinda learnt yoga and meditation from an early age, at Ashrams in India through her Anglo-Indian mother. Belinda teaches yoga in England and abroad and has a British Wheel of Yoga teaching qualification. Contact Belinda by:
Tel: 07985 057273
Email: belee@hotmail.com
or through the British Wheel.

ACKNOWLEDGEMENTS
Special thanks are due to Therese Diaz for help with photography.

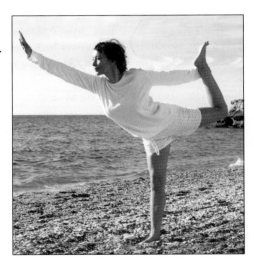

Other titles in the series

- **Understanding Acupressure**
- **Understanding Acupuncture**
- **Understanding The Alexander Technique**
- **Understanding Aloe Vera**
- **Understanding Aromatherapy**
- **Understanding Bach Flower Remedies**
- **Understanding The Bowen Technique**
- **Understanding Craniosacral Therapy**
- **Understanding Echinacea**
- **Understanding Evening Primrose**
- **Understanding Fish Oils**
- **Understanding Garlic**
- **Understanding Ginseng**
- **Understanding Head Massage**
- **Understanding Kinesiology**
- **Understanding Lavender**
- **Understanding Massage**
- **Understanding Pilates**
- **Understanding Reflexology**
- **Understanding Reiki**
- **Understanding St. John's Wort**
- **Understanding Shiatsu**

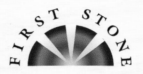

First published 2005 by First Stone Publishing
PO Box 8, Lydney, Gloucestershire, GL15 6YD

The contents of this book are for information only and are not intended as a substitute for appropriate medical attention. The author and publishers admit no liability for any consequences arising from following any advice contained within this book. If you have any concerns about your health or medication, always consult your doctor. The illustrations in this book are examples of yoga asanas only and are not intended to be copied by beginners. Consult your doctor before beginning any new exercise programme, particularly if you are pregnant, elderly or if you have any chronic or recurring physical conditions.

ISBN 1 904439 32 2

Printed and bound in Hong Kong through Printworks International Ltd.